WELCOME TO LONG-TERM CARE
PART 2

Welcome to Long-term Care, Part 2
Copyright © 2020 Bilquis Ali, RN

All rights reserved.

This book or any portion thereof may not be reproduced or used in any manner whatsoever without the express written permission of the publisher or author except for the use of brief quotations in a book review.

First Edition

WELCOME TO LONG-TERM CARE
PART 2

TABLE OF CONTENTS

Intro	1
Admissions	3
Incidents and Accidents	9
Pressure Ulcer/Injury	13
Education	17
Infection Prevention and Control	21
Customer Service	27
Care Planning	29
Activities	31
Policies/Procedures and Regulations	33
Anti-psychotics	35
QAPI	37
Survey Readiness	39
Year of the Nurse	41

WELCOME TO LONG-TERM CARE PART 2

Welcome back everyone to "Welcome To Long-Term Care" Book 2. This book we will focus on several topics and hopefully you will be able to bring it all together. I hope that you will be able to gain insight on how to improve the quality of care that you are providing by taking it a step further during your assessments. During this time also, think about how you can grow your team. Growing your team is crucial in improving outcomes and achieving Deficiency Free Surveys.

ADMISSIONS

How well are you investigating when you are admitting a new resident. Although facilities have a process for you to follow when completing an admission, how detailed are you with your process can essentially save you a lot of grief in the end. When you are admitting your resident, think with the end in mind. The end result being your survey. With that in mind, you will begin to get in the habit of being survey ready every day. For example, a preventative care plan isn't initiated upon admission and your resident now has a fall with injury possibly due to preventative measures not being implemented. So, when you are admitting think safety first.

This is my process:
I introduce myself to the resident. During my introduction, I am also assessing the resident orientation. I listen to their voice to assess for any weakness. I listen to how they

articulate their words and the excitement of the tone in their voice. This can indicate if the resident has accepted their new way of life, or if he/she requires support with adjusting to their new environment. Introduce their assigned nursing assistant during this time. This will allow him/her to have an immediate appointed staff member that they will be familiar with. This will also be an appropriate time to assess their skin if agreeable. Having two people assess is better than one. It's important to assess the skin as soon as possible. Delaying this process can result in an in house acquired pressure injury within hours, especially for a resident who is dependent upon staff to turn and reposition. Pressure ulcers/injury are a main topic in lawsuits in long-term care. Be proactive with identification and implementing preventative measures. Ensure your preventative measures are appropriate for the risk factors that are identified. Your risk factors stem from your Braden scale and underlying diagnosis. Document all of your findings in your admission assessment. Document that information in your care plan, and on your wound/skin sheet. Remember to also document bruises and their locations. If you don't document them on admission, I guarantee you that you will be investigating them in a few days when a staff member identifies this as a new area. If you observe your resident with dry and flaky skin, and are incontinent, implement a moisturizer and barrier cream. If your resident heels are soft and boggy, off load them to prevent further breakdown. Speak with the Physician and request an order for skin prep. What do their toes look like? Does he/she need to be placed on podiatrist list sooner rather than later? Does your resident have a history of falls? If so, do they happen at certain times of the day or when they are doing anything in particular? How are you going to keep him/her safe? We will discuss this later on more in depth. I then assess the oral cavity for pain. What does the tongue look like? Will this resident benefit from oral moisturizer? What is the resident oral hygiene routine? Does your resident have any problems chewing or swallowing? Your admission process can also be utilized as a time for education. Remember, they are new to you so you want to be able to obtain vital data that will allow you to provide him/her with the best care possible. Look at their fingers, do they have any clubbing of the fingers? Are their nails thick? Are their nails clean? Assess how they stand, and are they able to balance themselves? All of this is generally in your admission assessment. However, not everyone takes the time to appropriately assess these areas. The resident will have the best outcome when areas are identified in a timely manner and preventative measures are implemented. Preventative measures must be documented on the resident care plan. Assess vital signs and identify areas of concerns. It is a good practice to assess orthostatic blood pressures. This will guide you in implementing the most appropriate interventions to keeping your resident safe. Ask what time he/she morning and evening routine are? As stated previously, you want their plan of care to be specific to the resident, not to the facility. Residents need to feel like they have a homelike environment. They need to feel that they still have a form of control of their lives. Allowing them to be involved in their plan of will be beneficial.

What kind of environment do they like to be in? Often residents are paired with a roommate and they are not compatible. You can prevent a room move or grievance, if they are paired appropriately. Bowel health, another important area. The facility has their bowel protocol but find out what their pattern is. Your resident may tell you that they don't move their bowels daily. Assess for urinary pattern. You will implement your facility protocol for three-day bowel and bladder. Ask important questions such as nighttime urine, any frequency, does it interfere with sleep, any burning or leakage? Do they take any diuretics? All good data to implement in their care plan. What does their lower extremities look like? Are they edematous? Are they pitting or non-pitting? If edema is identified, this is good time to educate on ankle pumps and elevating their extremities. What do they feel like? Are they cold, warm or hot? Are they dry and discolored? How does he/she like to sleep at night? Do they like socks on. Are they able to wear non- skid slipper socks? Do they like the heat or air on? These are more topics again to implement the care plan.

Family/ social history: Family dynamics. How much fun this is. Not really. You will be amazed at how much valuable information you will retrieve from them. You will get to know more about why your resident needs to be in your facility. What was his/her routine at home. What did he/she do for a living? How were they in society and with other family members. For most families, admitting their loved one into a facility is by far the hardest decision of their life. For others it is a seemingly easy process. It is important that you obtain as much information as possible. You want to have one main contact person for your resident. Preferably one who is the power of attorney or resident representative. Family dynamics can become overwhelming for a facility especially when they do not have the appropriate contact person. Has your new resident been in the military or war at all? This is important because it will give you more ideas on the behaviors they may have or even if they may have suffered any type of trauma. If you identify that they have experienced any form of trauma, implement trauma informed care plan in implement interventions as appropriate.

If you are in the state of Pennsylvania, implement the POLST form and ensure that it is completed entirely. Completing this form should not be a rush discussion. Be sure that resident and resident representative understands the questions. Administer the first step of the PPD immunization and document it on the medication record and the immunization tab. Vaccinations should be addressed at this time as well. If it is flu season, offer and administer the flu vaccination. If they are appropriate to receive the pneumococcal vaccination, offer and administer and document this in the immunization tab. Ensure that you have signed consents from the resident and or the resident representative. Immunizations are a sub-standard quality care citation. Be proactive in addressing this area on admission.

Review the medications with him/her and find out again the routine that they had at home. Were they compliant with taking their medications? If not, find out why? What do you need to provide to them to meet their needs? Review diagnosis and introduce them to their new environment. Before you leave the room, introduce him/her to their roommate and ask them if there is anything else that you can do for them? Ensure that the call bell is in reach and that the resident is able to demonstrate proper use of it.

When you are admitting your resident, pull your policy for your admission process and ensure you are adhering to it. This is a great way to be and stay prepared. This is the best way to improve outcomes for your residents and your facilities. Stay ready so, you don't have to get ready.

INCIDENTS AND ACCIDENTS

The inability of following through to ensure that the process is not only complete, but interventions are appropriate. Often when an incident occurs, staff may not implement an immediate intervention. More importantly the appropriate intervention. The intervention must connect to the root cause in order to be effective. This is not to say that another episode won't occur. However, it is to say that the same exact scenario is less likely to occur and if and when it does, then we need to go back and collaborate to come up with the best solution. With that being said, it requires staff to dig deeper to identify the most appropriate intervention.

For example. Your resident has a fall out of bed. Your witness statements all state that the resident was trying to go to the bathroom. The staff member places an intervention to say, educate the resident to ring call bell for assistance. There are several concerns with this intervention. First, the intervention to ring call bell for assistance should be standard for all residents that are appropriate. You later identify that the resident is moderately impaired and therefore, cannot be educated but rather encouraged. The concern with this, due to the resident memory, he/she may not remember to ring the call bell for assistance.

How could you attempt to identify the most appropriate root cause? Several areas could be addressed.
First, did anyone interview the resident? If so, what did the statement say? What is the resident BIMS and is the resident a credible? Although, a resident may be deemed moderately impaired, they may have the ability to answer simple and direct questions. If you find this is the case, ask simple one worded question to obtain information from the resident. Were there any areas that stood out to you that would assist you in identifying the root cause. Second, did the staff re-enact the fall to justify if it correlates with the statement from the resident and the staff witness statements? Third, medication review to see if the resident takes any diuretics later in the day that would cause frequent urination, or what time does the resident get bedtime meds and or snack and liquids that would cause the resident with frequent trips to the bathroom. Remember, to be as specific as possible to the resident pattern, not your own. Did this resident have any other falls that are similar to the same scenario as well as the intervention that were implemented? Did vitals show any changes in orthostatic pressures?

These are just some factors to consider when an accident occurs. From there, review the previous falls. Identify any areas that have the same root cause and intervention. What this will do is bring insight on identifying the frequency of these occurrences. It will also help you identify what interventions were effective. If interventions are no longer effective, update care plan accordingly.

Incidents and accidents can occur in any area of your facility. It is everyone responsibility to ensure the safety of resident and staff. The more your staff are educated on processes the better outcome you have for all. Another example is the famous medication not available. Many do not think that is an issue. It is a major issue. What is the process that you have in place to ensure medications are available at all times? I understand if you receive a new admission late in the evening and the medications didn't arrive in time. If that is the case, have your pharmacy company contact a local pharmacy to have them deliver the medications that are needed. It is a good practice to identify what medications are utilized most utilized most and add them to your emergency box. I've seen this happen many of times. You want to meet the needs of the residents at all times. This will prevent having a delay in medications being administered.

Incidents can occur by not following the resident plan of care. The resident plan of care needs to be clear so that there is no confusion in regard to what is to be provided. State the facts only. What does your staff need to now in order to effectively take care of Jane?

A few other areas to review and ensure processes are in place are your smoking residents, resident to resident altercations, residents who utilize side rails, and unlocked medication carts. I will always be a fan of rounding. Rounding can assist you in improving your outcomes in those areas.

PRESSURE ULCERS/INJURY

One of the areas that did not want to receive a citation for are pressure ulcer/injury. For starters, it was because I took it personally as a leader of a facility if a resident sustained a pressure injury or if they were admitted with an injury and it declined. There are few residents that are at a higher risk for pressure injury and may sustain one. Then there are those that are unavoidable which are very few if this is the case, make sure your physician has it documented as such. What can you do to prevent a pressure injury? Let's take it back to our admission assessment. This is crucial to know what preventative measures are needed to prevent pressure injury. If and when an injury has occurred, what process do you have in place to address all concerns. The questionnaire that I created below is a guide to assist the nurse with the thought process to meet the needs of the resident. Review it and see if I covered anything that you may not have. I'm not

Welcome to Long-term Care

PRESSURE ULCER QUESTIONNAIRE

Resident Name:_____Admission Date:_____

INQUIRY	YES	NO	COMMENTS / CONCERNS
Diagnosis that could attribute to skin ulcer?			
Medications that could attribute to skin ulcer?			
Braden upon admission?			
Previous braden?			
Current braden?			
Did resident mobility decline?			
What is the resident bed mobility?			
What was resident weight on admission?			
Most current weight?			
Did resident have any weight loss?			
What is resident diet?			
Meal intake?			
Most recent note from dietician?			
Any dietician concerns?			
What recommendations does the dietician have to promote wound healing?			
Does resident utilize dentures?			
Any concerns with mouth pain?			
Last visit with dentist?			
Were any concerns on dental form?			
What is the resident most recent BIMS?			
Does this resident have any behaviors?			
Does this resident refuse care?			
Are these refusals in resident care plan and have been addressed?			
Is the resident bedridden, wheelchair bound or ambulatory?			
If and what is resident's physical therapy plan?			
Is the resident incontinent of bowel and bladder?			
How often is resident showered?			
When was resident last showered?			

©2020 Bilquis Ali All Rights Reserved.

Welcome to Long-term Care

Resident Name:_____ Admission Date:_____

INQUIRY	YES	NO	COMMENTS / CONCERNS
Had the resident had any medical illness that would cause a decline?			
Date of pressure ulcer?			
Stage of pressure ulcer?			
Witness statements for 72 hours prior to identification?			
Was a root cause identified?			
Were interventions in place PRIOR to pressure ulcer?			
What were those interventions?			
What intervention implemented for new ulcer?			
Was MD and resident representative made aware?			
Any new orders from MD?			
Could this pressure ulcer been avoided?			
When was the last visit to MD?			
Did MD have any concerns documented or any declines?			
Was pain management implemented for this resident?			
What is the treatment order for the wound?			
Is the order complete with appropriate treatment, location and frequency of treatment?			
Is wound documented on skin/wound sheet?			
Is it updated in care plan?			
Was resident representative updated on new interventions and order?			
How did resident representative respond to the pressure ulcer on resident?			
What process will you put in place to monitor and measure this wound?			
Initiate therapy screen			

Once you have answered the questions: ❑ Complete an IDT note that this event was reviewed.
If this wound could have been avoided:
❑ Initiate a Performance Improvement Plan.
❑ Identify any other residents that are at an increase risk for pressure ulcers to ensure interventions are in place.
❑ Complete a full house skin sweep.
❑ Review facility treatment policy and dressing change.
❑ Begin to competency nurses on treatment for proper technique to promote wound healing.
❑ Schedule a meeting a your MDS coordinator.

©2020 Bilquis Ali All Rights Reserved.

stating I have all the answers. I am stating, I have fifteen years of experience and I will forever be a student. I continuously learn to improve myself so that I may assist those in need. I enjoy learning how to improve my skills daily.

EDUCATION

How important is education to you? How often do you educate not only your staff but more importantly yourself? Think about that and think about the amount of incident and accidents that you have acquired. Has the lack of education attributed to these incidents occurring? Review your orientation process. What does that look like? How does your nurse educator interact with the employees? Are your employees engaged? Orientation is crucial for new employees. It is imperative to set the expectations in that setting. Review policies and procedures. This will improve the quality of care for your residents. Education cannot be a read and sign. It should include a return demonstration and test at the end to ensure that the employees have comprehended and understand the material. It should be informative, fun and include scenarios. You will have more participation from staff in this manner and they won't feel like they are being put on the spot. It is also important to identify learning barriers. If you identified that they don't understand something, what other measures will you take to help them understand? Do you merely say, you will get it in due time, or do you take the time now? Have you identified why they don't understand it? Do they have a learning barrier or is it a behavior? Be aware of the differences. If it is a behavior concern, it will take countless re-enforcement of proper practice. Habits are hard to break. It is important for staff to understand policies and procedures are in place to protect the resident and them. They do not want to end up in court for not following it and having a major injury. Be the change, and part of the solution to create a safe environment. If possible, provide education that are set up like a classroom and have the staff take notes. They need to understand that education is important. If possible, have it set up quarterly with your mannequin and they can perform return demonstration on the mannequin, and this will allow them time to ask questions? Another idea for new nurses and new hires is to order the candy medication packs. Have medication administration records and observe them with administering medication with the mannequin. Allow them to practice before they work on the floor. Have different routes to allow you to assess technique. It's a good idea to practice in the classroom to assess a baseline and areas for opportunity. Take the time to provide them the tools that they need before they work the floor. I know with the pandemic and the staffing crisis; this may sound impossible. However, residents deserve to be provided the best care with best practice. This will also improve staff confidence in their role. Any opportunity you have to educate, EDUCATE. There is no such thing as too much education.

INFECTION PREVENTION AND CONTROL

I must admit, I loved infection prevention and control until COVID 19.

I'm sure by now, you have learned much more about the virus and ways of decreasing the spread. I was confused with the Yellow Zone. I could give two shits about that zone. I wanted green and red. PERIOD. It became so overwhelming deciding who went where. Now that the cases are decreasing, it is much more simplified. But I am telling you. I am not looking forward to flu season and this damn virus. This is going to increase our testing because of the similarities between the two. So, make sure you have the process in place. Make sure you are tracking on your line listings and reporting as appropriate. Some facilities are opening up to which I think is great. Our residents need to able to see their families. I have noticed so many residents with increased behaviors as well as depression due to the lack of visitations from their family.

How can you tell the nurses that we can't hug our residents anymore? That was so difficult. They are our family as well. How can you tell the demented resident that they have to stay in their room, when they don't understand it?

The term recently changed from infection control and prevention to now infection prevention and control. The goal of course is always to prevent. What does that mean for you? At this time, no one can afford to get this citation. However, it will be an easy citation to get if your facility has issues with the mere basics of infection prevention such as hand hygiene, not carrying linen in your hands that is soiled, having personal food on medication cart, food at the nurse's station. These are the basics so be mindful and observant of these areas. Increase your rounding now before survey. I talked a lot about rounding in book one, and it didn't change. The best way to prevent is to know. Know what staff are doing on the floors so you can educate and correct. Remember habits are hard to break. Remember how many times you wanted to make a change such as a diet, yet you kept eating snickers, that's how your staff feel. Most have the intention of doing better but because it is a habit, they have to repeatedly be told about it at the time it occurs, not after you observed them completing. If you observe them doing it and not interrupt the thought process while it is happening, it will still manifest as if they are doing nothing wrong.

How do you track your infections? How do you know what areas of opportunity you need to focus on? I myself am a fan of mapping. I enjoy being able to know where the bacteria it is and where it went and track the staff that might have increased the spread. I enjoy antibiotic stewardship program. It is important that you adhere to the antibiotic stewardship program. Ensure you have proper documentation such as a chest-x-ray, labs including a culture and sensitivity report prior to antibiotics being ordered. Your physicians are aware of this process, yet not all of them follow it. Now if your resident is symptomatic, then that is a different scenario. Keep in mind to remember to assess symptoms prior to see if it meets the reporting requirements if you have them for you state. If you aren't familiar with McGeer Criteria for Long-Term Care, I recommend you reviewing this tool and meet with your leadership team and incorporate it into your process. An important factor of having control of your facility from an infection prevention aspect is to have someone on each shift playing a role in it. For example, educate your evening nurses on how to read the culture reports and complete the infection sheet. Educate them on the policies for precautions. Someone else besides the infection prevention nurse and nurse director needs to be aware of infection prevention. This will decrease system failure as well. When you have your infection meeting, make sure you have someone from housekeeping, especially if you have outbreaks. This is a team effort to contain it. Not just nursing.

We are now in flu season. The Covid 19 rates are now increasing again in some areas. Some facilities are opening up to visitors now. I am going to be honest; I am concerned. Concerned with this season battling both viruses. Influenza and Covid. In the planner Welcome to Long-Term Care, in the month of September tab, I had it labeled, "Did you start getting flu consents". I wanted facilities to start mailing and calling families to get residents consents for flu vaccination. They will need it for sure this season. Also, pneumococcal vaccinations need to be up to date. If your resident would be diagnosed with pneumonia, did you offer them the vaccination prior. Prevention is key. Remember that Influenza and Pneumococcal immunizations are substandard quality care. Make sure you have a solid process with this area and are adhering to your facility policy.

What are your thoughts about visitation? I am excited for the residents to be re-united with their loved ones. They all need it. As the leader, you need to ensure their safety while visiting. Make sure your signs are up for flu season even if you have no visitations. Some facilities have started being surveyed, and you don't want to have that as a mention in your survey.

Housekeeping is a key role in the decrease the spread of infections. It is even more vital than what we think. Think of all the surfaces bacteria harbor. Now imagine if these areas aren't being cleaned effectively. What do you think will happen? While you are sitting around looking for the root cause, the root cause may be the house keeping. Be observant of how they clean and the pattern that they clean. They should be cleaning the same as we do. From clean to dirty not dirty to clean. Any rooms that are isolated should have another cleaning schedule. Meet with your housekeeper daily, especially if you have an outbreak. Find out what is the plan in place to assist you in preventing the spread. One department can't do it alone. As always, it takes a team effort to have the best outcomes. Once you have established a routine with the department, you should be able to notice a decrease. If you don't, then you need to go back and identify the root cause of the spread. It can be anyone, so don't take it personal. Just work together as a team to resolve it. Bring the issue to meeting and meet daily and also monthly at your QAPI meeting. Other areas to be aware of in regard to housekeeping is to make sure the housekeeping carts are off the unit when the trays come up to floor from the kitchen. I observed this many of times. It is an unnecessary infection control citation. Again, you can work with all departments to put together a schedule to make sure they are following processes. It might take a while if they aren't used to doing it. Stay with it, it will get better.

While meals are being served, take advantage of this time to observe practices that break infection prevention and control such as not washing hands between feeding a resident and getting another tray. Make sure staff aren't touching resident's food with bare hands. Small simple tasks that you can observe and correct immediately if observed. Another area to review is refrigerators in the pantry and if the resident has their own refrigerator. As much as I am an advocate for residents' rights, for the love of GOD, I despise the refrigerator in their room. If you don't have a process to ensure that their refrigerator is being checked EVERYDAY!! Then please get one and make sure you have a backup person for when the routine person is off. As far as the refrigerators on the unit, I haven't worked one place where we just can't seem to decide who tasks is it to complete. Housekeeping always says nursing, nursing says housekeeping, and someone yells dietary. Someone needs to take ownership for it. Again, a team effort for the best outcome. All items in the refrigerator MUST be DATED. NO EXCEPTIONS. If it belongs to a resident, the resident name must be on it as well as the date and remember the THREE-DAY RULE. Anything after that DISCARD.

CUSTOMER SERVICE

This is a topic that I just can't talk about ENOUGH. Yes, we know that our residents and their families our customers. However, there is one very important customer that you can't survive without. Those customers are your staff. I am a big advocate for staff appreciation. When you appreciate them, they perform better? When they are happy, your residents are happy. Yes, some leaders will say, well they were hired to do a job. I say and so were you. As the leader of the building you need to make sure that they will return to work. Employee retention is a good place to start. No staff member wakes up and says, "I want to go to work and do a poor job". However, depending on the type of environment they walked in when they arrived at work, can change everything. If they arrive to work and are immediately staff challenged, and given orders before they could even clock in, is a problem. Be proactive instead of reactive. Have a plan in place. Train your staff to have a plan in place on what do if there are challenges. Staff appreciation goes a long way. It's not just showering them with gifts, but it is to genuinely want to know how they're doing and what could the facility do as a whole to head in the right direction. Remember, as the leader, you won't, and you don't have all the answers. If you do, think you have all the answers, your staff will become silent. They will no longer provide you with feedback. You will learn very quickly. And they will say, I tried to tell you, but you didn't listen. So, listen to them, embrace their ideas. Let them know that you will include them in making decisions that will directly impact them. After all, the decisions you make will not affect you, rather it will affect them. Again, don't ask your staff to do anything that you wouldn't do. When nurse's week and nursing assistant week arrives, go all out for them. Never like before, they need to be appreciated for nurse's week and

CARE PLANNING

nursing assistant week 2021.

Care plans should look like your resident. It should be individualized to the resident, and should include diagnosis, preferences and what staff need to know to care for the resident. If the resident doesn't get out of bed until 9 am and wants breakfast at 9:30, then their care plan should reflect that. If the resident spits out his/her medications, that should be documented in the care plan. If they like wearing shorts in the winter, add it to their care plan. Your resident doesn't like to shower because they were scolded in hot water, but they will allow you to provide them a bed bath. That is what your care plan needs to say and add a trauma informed care plan because you have now identified trauma. Think of your care plan as your road map to provide the best care possible to your resident. It doesn't need to have 100 problems and 100 interventions if you aren't utilizing it.

The more it is individualized and specific to the resident, the better outcomes you will have.

Important information to have in place, are preventive care plans. As I stated earlier, the goal is always to prevent, this means having the care plan in place for skin, fall, pain and ADLs. What about your diagnosis? If you are treating it, then it needs to be in the care plan. Quarterly, you will have a care plan meeting, take advantage of this time and thoroughly review and resolve any care plans and interventions that are no longer appropriate. While you are reviewing the care plan, make sure that the code status is accurate and up to date. Don't assume that the resident or resident representative didn't change their mind. Address any psych diagnosis with social services and make sure that interventions are appropriate if any behaviors are observed. There is never too much information in a care plan if it accurate and individualized to your resident. It becomes ineffective when interventions are put in place that are not appropriate.

ACTIVITIES

Let me just start by saying, thank you to all our activities staff. This pandemic required them to think outside the box to ensure the residents needs were being met. This was absolutely heartbreaking, and residents didn't understand what was going on and why couldn't they come out of their room and why couldn't their families come to see them. I mean absolutely heart breaking. Activities play a major role in a resident's well-being. It is vital for most to be active and engaged. It also improves their quality of life. Think back to the admission process, when you are gathering data from your resident / resident representative. For example, my father he is a workaholic. I always tell him you are going to be a difficult nursing home resident. He is always busy. He doesn't know what rest is. He works every day, drives long distances, his sleep pattern is that he wakes up around 4-5 every morning. What will his plan of care look like from activities perspective? You were just informed on how active and independent he is. Now imagine being confined to one location, with no vehicle and someone telling him to go back to bed when he wakes up every day at this time for prayer. This is why it is important to gather as much information from your admission assessment so your resident needs can be met. The activities director would have to know this information to make sure he will be going out on all the outings and talking to families and making prayer services. You want to promote your resident's independence and improve the quality of life as much as you can. I will hopefully have the privilege of caring for my parents at home as I did for my grandparents. It is such a blessing. However, not everyone has this ability which is why we need to gather as much information as possible to ensure the best quality of life that they can have. If you have younger residents, you want to make sure that your activities are appropriate for their age group, not he seniors unless they are agreeable to it. They maybe into social media and enjoy being on the computer and going on frequent trips. You want to make sure you gage their plan of care to be specific for them.

POLICIES/PROCEDURES AND REGULATIONS

Policies are in place for a reason. You shouldn't function without them. It is imperative that your staff have access to facilities policies 24/7. They need to be able to use it as a resource. If you do not educate them on it, they will never learn. They have to be able to function independently. You want your team to make this part of their language. I would often get teased by my staff because I was always talking about policies, procedures and regulations. That is how I reviewed my clinical process by identifying what possible citations we would get by not adhering to a policy. Every building that I enter, I give them a copy of F-tag list and show them how to get to a regulation and show them how to use Appendix PP Guidance for Surveyors. Wherever I go, my regulation book goes, and I study my regulation book like I am studying for an exam. I mentioned earlier that I am a career learner. If I don't know the answer, I know how to find it. Provide your staff the tools that they need to be successful. What I have found is that when staff do not know the policy, the work blindly assuming that what they are doing is correct and that is not the case. Can you imagine having a building of nurses and they all think like you? It is not impossible. I have been called on my days off and if something happened, they would say what would Bilquis do? They would tell me I would stalk them in their mind. They were learning. That made me feel good. That is what you want. No one wants to come to work and say I want to do a poor job. Staff want to do good. Support them and give them what they need so they can. Never talk down to them if they do not know something. That will cause them to make many mistakes and cover it up all because of the fear of embarrassment.

ANTIPSYCHOTICS

Antipsychotics MUST have an approved diagnosis in order to receive them. If they do not have an approved diagnosis and have not been trialled on a different medication, then the physician needs to do so. Every day, someone should review these medications to ensure they have the appropriate diagnosis and if not, what is the plan to either get the diagnosis or attempt a GDR. Remember they MUST be an APPROVED diagnosis. Dementia is not an approved diagnosis for an antipsychotic medication. You should facilitate a monthly behavior meeting at minimum. Weekly, if you have a large facility. This meeting should also include your psych consultant and pharmacy consultant if possible and social services. Have this meeting and be creative with it. Review the care plan and make sure that it is appropriate and specific for the resident. The behaviors that the resident exhibits must be in the care plan. It is pointless to have these meetings and not review key components. Meet with your psych consultant if a mediation was ordered and do not utilize the appropriate diagnosis. I have seen this happen too many times. Not all consultants are familiar with long-term care regulations. It is important that you explain it to them and that they understand it. You don't want to get an unnecessary citation.

QAPI

This is the meeting that brings it all together. It is imperative that you take this meeting seriously. Issues that you find in your facility are merely opportunities for improvement. This is the place to collectively meet as a team to come up with solutions and track and trend to have the best outcome. For example, any concerns that you have in your clinical process, you can initiate a performance improvement plan and write out a performance improvement plan and discuss that data monthly in this meeting. It's good to get feedback especially from your medical director. Your medical director should always be aware of what areas of concerns you have in your building, this way they can also provide feedback on how to improve the process. This meeting should be monthly. Quarterly, your medical director, pharmacy consultant, lab consultant and diagnostics, should attend. Take pride in the areas of opportunity and create the facility you want. QAPI meetings and performance improvements plans are beneficial only if you work the process. It is pointless to identify areas and not carry them out. Always celebrate the wins regardless how small when you notice an improvement.

The most important lesion I want you to take from this is INVESTIGATE, INVESTIGATE, INVESTIGATE. Do not just accept things for what they are. Every opportunity that you identify will have a root cause. You must identify it. Notice how I change the language from problems to opportunity. When we think of them as problems, that is just how we treat them and become frustrated. When we think of them as opportunity, it forces us to think of the outcome we will reach. In the event that you identify an urgent concern, initiate an ADHOC and inform everyone what happened and what is the plan to correct it. This could be on a resident who might have eloped from your facility. You would then initiate this meeting and do a house audit to identify the root cause of why and how it happened. Education must be included in this and you should try to get 100% with education staff on the new process.

SURVEY READINESS

This is the one area that must be taken very seriously. In the first book, I talked about being survey ready every day. If you get in the habit of thinking like this, you will become this. It is important that the 802 and 672 are updated at a minimum weekly. That means, in morning clinical while you are reviewing new admissions, someone is updating that information into these forms. Along with these documents, make sure that reportable events are completed with statements, care plan, orders, face sheet, neuro checks, skin sheets and incident report. Keep printed the three latest PB22 that was reported and ensure these are completed. Meet with my medical records department for closed charts and review information and make sure discharged charts are completed. With closed charts, you want to make sure that your medication requisition form is completed and personal belongings sheet. Whoever is responsible for infection prevention, ensure that all antibiotics sheets are updated, and that infection mapping and line listing are updated. Ensure you have a current copy of all pressure wound tracking sheets. If it was an in house acquired, make sure you have an incident report that is completed, and care plan is updated. It is a good practice to track Foley catheters, central lines, dialysis, peg tubes, anything that would be considered a quality of care area. We do track this in the Welcome To Long-Term Care Planner. This may seem like a lot of work. It is. However, once you get in the habit of doing it, it will become second nature for you and your team. Do not just prepare your survey binder when you are in your survey window. Have your survey binder completed all the time. *"It is better to be prepared for an opportunity and not have one than to have an opportunity and not be prepared."* (Whitney M. Young).

When the Department of Health arrives to your facility whether it is routine or a complaint visit, show them who you are by being prepared. You Got This!

THE YEAR OF THE NURSE

This is what they are saying about us. I don't know about you, but I am over it and want it to go away like the minute it came out. I remember it like yesterday literally. I remember putting everything into place on March 14th. What I wouldn't know is that my world would be a nightmare. I think the most frustrating part for me was the amount of times the questions and answers changed. I felt very incompetent as a nurse and even more as a leader. How the hell was I the nurse leader of the facility keep my resident and staff safe when the government had no clue what to do either. It was so overwhelming and frustrating. But, like everything, I researched, and I read and read and read some more to still felt like I had no idea of what was going on. I remember vividly educating my staff over and over and over again on the process we put in place. I went to work every morning at

4:30 to do all the check in for staff. I made videos and posted them on my Facebook page because I wanted everyone to be informed as much as possible. The sad part is, the government still was in the unknown on how to contain this virus. So, I continued to go in and my staff continued to show up. I was so grateful to them and very appreciative for them taking it seriously and asking questions and taking notes. It is the part that made me keep going. We were family, we worked hard together and stayed together. Our first case, we were all nervous. I took the care of the first resident. Never ask you staff to do anything that you wouldn't do. I felt it was my duty to lead by example and that is what I did. What I didn't know was how fast the medical status would change. I mean I am staring IV lines, placing oxygen, calling doctors for orders and assessing continuously. My staff was right there with me. We were a united front to ensure the safety of our residents. There would be many sleepless nights, early mornings. Many days without having clinical because our focus was this virus. At this point, nothing else seemed to matter. Months went by and the cases grew and grew. Now my staff were getting sick too. So, what happens then. You have to bring agency in to meet the needs of the residents. It was the first time that I have had to use agency and I was proud of it. I was grateful that they came to help us. I thanked them every day for coming in. They were putting their lives on the line as well. We all did. That is the world of nursing. While many were saying, well this is what we signed up for? Shame on them. We signed up to care for those whom no longer could care for themselves and our goal is to improve the quality of life. We like everyone else, wanted to make it home to our families too. Was that too much to ask? Apparently, it was. We worked countless days and night with no days off to ensure the safety of our residents. If we wouldn't do it then who will? That's right. No one. We were now the ones who were saving the world. How about that. It took many lives to be lost to the virus for us to be praised for what we were doing. Cases were up in an astronomical rate. My thought was, the focus should have been on nursing homes rather than hospitals because our population is much more in terms of numbers. That wasn't the case. It wasn't until there were massive death rates that it was decided that we need help. What would that help look like? It would look like nurses being able to practice in other states due to the crisis. My thought was why would we have to have a pandemic in order for this to come about? The now laymen person can take an 8-hour training course and be able to work as a temporary nursing assistant. Staffing was in crisis in places before pandemic in many areas. Why, again would it take a pandemic for this to happen. As time went on, rates continued to rise. In May, I contracted the virus. I remember going to the store and feeling a migraine coming on. I said to myself "oh goodness I'm getting a migraine". I got back home and felt a little chilly and thought oh, but it subsided. The next morning, I text my team and let them know that I was going to be a few hours late because I couldn't shake this migraine. None of us thought anything, because I would get migraines routinely. I text an hour later, and I had a temperature. I thought oh shit I have this virus. I went and got tested and got my results the next day. I was positive. I had every system and it was awful. I couldn't move and I was scared for my life. So scared that I called my insurance company to make changes to my policies. I called my oldest son and told him about my insurance policy. Can you imagine having to have this conversation with your child. I needed to ensure that he knew the plan. My mother would facetime me several times a day and I had to lie and tell her I was okay when I wasn't. I couldn't tell anyone in my family that I was scared for my life. I was away from my family and I had not seen my children in now months. A few months went by and I recovered, I had lost 15 lbs. And it took a good couple of months for my lungs to feel almost resolved. It is a time that I will never forget. That the world would never forget…

This book is part two. I hope you enjoy it as you did with book one. Again, my method is informative and to the point. This book is written off of 15 years of experience in long-term care.

Feel free to follow me on IG@welcometolongtermcare.

Link Tree: https://linktr.ee/bilquis
My website is Welcometolong-termcare.com and email consultant@welcometolong-termcare.com.

I provide a survey preparation course to assist you in achieving a Deficiency Free Survey.

One person can't do it alone, but together we can make a difference.

Made in the USA
Middletown, DE
22 September 2024

60862997R00031